High Risk: Truth, Lies, & Birth

Leigh Fransen

www.honestmidwife.com

At Least As Safe

The young, eager couple sat across from me in my living room. The woman, her straight blond hair parted in the middle, was noticeably pregnant. Excited, a little nervous, they asked questions about me: Where had I gone to school? How many births had I attended? What kinds of medical equipment did I have, and what kinds of birth experiences could I support?

I answered them reassuringly, in the practiced style of a seasoned salesperson. My father had sold many products in his time: fancy windows, expensive decks, elaborate log homes. I inherited my power of persuasion from him. I told the couple about my schooling, my experience, and my philosophy of care. Yes, I was well-trained in water birth; yes, they could refuse any shots for their newborn. I knew the answers they wanted to hear, and I was happy to deliver all the right ones. There seemed little doubt that they would agree: I would be their midwife and manage their birth at the out-of-hospital birth center I co-owned.

One question, tacked on at the end, caught me only a little off-guard. The woman hesitated a little and asked, "And… this is, um, *safe*… right?"

I breathed deep, and replied with the most honest answer I knew to give: "It's as safe as life gets. Nothing is risk-free. Driving down the highway to get here was not risk-free. Many studies have shown that birth outside of the hospital is *at least as safe* as birth in the hospital for low-risk women like you. And I'm very conservative. I won't hesitate to take you to the hospital if I get concerned about anyone's safety." Yes, I was prepared to handle any and every eventuality.

I was hired. It was 2009, and I was on the cusp of a very successful stint as a birth center owner and licensed midwife, credentialed by the state of South Carolina. It would be years before I would truly confront the underlying deception of the answer I gave that day.

A Midwife is Born

Although nonhospital births (births that occur in a home, free-standing birth center, or other location that is not inside or attached to a hospital) account for less than 2% of births in the United States, they have substantially increased since 2004. In 2013, the last year for which the CDC has released birth statistics, 1.42% of U.S. births for which birthplace was reported were not in a hospital, up from 0.87% only 9 years earlier in 2004.

I first entered the world of natural birth when I was pregnant with my first child in 2002. Having attended a breastfeeding support group, I was invited to attend a local "Parent Topic Night" about doulas. Doulas are women who provide professional birth support to women giving birth in any setting. The people I met were incredibly kind and very interested in me. I decided to hire a doula (I ended up hiring two) and had a natural, drug-free birth in a local hospital. The experience was such a good one, so much better than I had ever imagined it could be, that I decided to become a doula myself.

After attending a small handful of births as a doula, I decided that it wasn't for me. I didn't enjoy feeling as if I had no power to really help these women achieve a natural birth. I felt like they were at the mercy of the hospital, and it could be a very hostile environment; doctors and nurses pushed interventions and medications even when they seemed to me to be unnecessary and counterproductive. I decided that if I really wanted to make a difference, I would need to become a midwife.

By the time I was due to have my second child, I was enrolled in a midwifery school accredited by the state of Florida. I gave birth in the same birth center where I was trained, one of the busiest midwife-owned birth centers in the country. I graduated after three years of hard work, having excelled in my classes and having attended over 150 births, and thus earning an occupational associate's degree in midwifery. I moved my family up to South Carolina where I proceeded to obtain my midwifery license and open my own birth center, with the partnership of three other South Carolina midwives.

In 2008, former talk-show host Ricki Lake released *The Business of Being Born*. This brilliantly done, emotionally compelling documentary helped propel nonhospital birth into the public consciousness. Lake has written about her own influence: "Every day women stop me on the street to share stories of their safe, successful, meaningful births. Many say they felt 'in the dark' about their options until seeing *The Business of Being Born.*" As 25% owner and marketing manager of the Carolina Community Maternity Center in Fort Mill, South Carolina, from 2009-2013, I made this documentary part of our regular free childbirth classes for the community. By the time the credits rolled, I was almost guaranteed new clients, freshly converted from planning a hospital birth to planning a birth center birth with me or one of my partners as midwife.

"Doing My Research"

It seems a popular notion that once you have read enough material from any source to make up your mind about a topic, you can declare, "I have done my research," and rest assured that your opinion is at least as valid as anyone else's. I felt I had "done my research" regarding the safety of nonhospital birth when I opted to give birth to my second daughter in a warm bathtub at a freestanding birth center, attended by two licensed midwives and two student midwives. It was an extraordinary experience that was captured, with my approval, by the Discovery Health channel for international broadcast. I wanted to be on the show to help demonstrate that natural birth with midwives was a lovely experience to aspire to, in hopes that other women would dare to believe that they too could have a wonderful birth experience. My motives, both in choosing the birth center and in agreeing to the filming, were largely the same: I wanted an amazing experience, and I wanted to share it with the world. I wanted to avoid medical intervention and achieve something that many women seemed to think was outrageously difficult. I knew my baby would be fine, never doubted for a moment she would be, and she was. This was my experience, and I wanted to help others have the same sort of marvelous and enviable start to their parenting journey.

Fast-forward almost a decade, and I'm sitting in a university library. I have decided that it is high time that I did the legwork and read for myself the scientific literature regarding the safety of giving birth in a nonhospital setting. After years of assuring others of what "the studies show," I wanted to do more than rely on others' interpretations. I knew I wasn't the first (or the most qualified) person to ever undertake this, but I could represent your average midwife who always took other people's word that the safety of what I was doing was backed by evidence. I had to admit that regardless of how many books, blogs, websites, and Wikipedia articles I had previously read, I had never actually "done my research."

I began in familiar territory, the website of the Midwives Alliance of North America (MANA.org). On this site there is a button titled "Research," and it leads to an extensive collection of the studies that MANA has determined builds the case that nonhospital birth with a midwife is safe. MANA has categorized the research into sections A-F, Section A containing the "best available studies on planned home birth and maternal fetal outcomes." Section B contains "studies exhibiting problems with the design, analysis or reporting" and so on, with the evidence becoming weaker as the letters progress. I opened up Section A and noted that it was divided into five tiers and included a total of 24 studies. Perfect! MANA had provided me with the 24 best studies to prove the safety of home birth. I spent the next several hours using my university library (and helpful librarians) to track down every one of these 24 studies and print them out, filling a large 3-ring binder with my efforts.

Shades of guilt danced in the back of my head: shouldn't I have done this years ago? Perhaps before I decided to actually give birth to my own child in a bathtub in a residential neighborhood in Miami? Possibly during my years as a student of midwifery? Maybe before I had assured scores of women that "research showed" giving birth at my birth center was as safe as any hospital? I cleared my head to focus on the task at hand. The research was all here in front of me now. I sat down with my giant binder of studies, a cup of coffee, and a handful of pens and highlighters. I had a long day ahead of me. I began at the beginning of MANA's list.

Section I: Meta-analyses and Systematic Reviews

Olsen & Clausen: The first study listed, by Olsen and Clausen, was from 2012 and was published in the Cochrane Database of Systematic Reviews. It purported to be a systematic review of randomized controlled trials of home birth. This seemed to me to be a curious and difficult way to study home birth, as it would require randomly selecting women to give birth at home. Although randomized controlled trials are considered the "gold standard" of research, how could one ethically assign women to birth at home or hospital? I didn't have to wonder long: the systematic review only determined that there are no usable randomized controlled clinical trials. They only were able to find one study that fit their criteria for inclusion, and the sample size of eleven women was too small to be of any statistical use to anyone.

Leslie & Romano: The second study listed was a systematic review of nonhospital birth studies by Leslie and Romano, published in the *Journal of Perinatal Education* in 2007. Now, I do think it is important to note that the *Journal of Perinatal Education* is the official "journal" of Lamaze International. This means that it is sponsored by an organization whose bread and butter is based on natural childbirth education. This does not mean they are incapable of publishing valid findings, but it is prudent to be aware of the money behind a publication when evaluating a study.

The Leslie and Romano study found that nonhospital birth results in far fewer interventions, such as cesarean sections, use of intravenous fluids, and use of medical pain control. They cite three studies in their finding that perinatal mortality[1] rates are "similar" to that of the hospital: Gulbranson (1997), Janssen et al (2002), and Olsen (1997). The Janssen study is covered under Section III, discussed later in this paper. The Gulbranson study was conducted in New Zealand and determined a perinatal death rate of 2.97 per thousand; I clearly needed to find out if this was truly "similar" to hospital rates, so I highlighted this number and made a mental note to come back to it.

Olsen: The third study used by Leslie and Romano for perinatal mortality comparison is also the last study in section I: Olsen from 1997, "Meta-analysis of the safety of home birth." This is the second listing from Olsen in the first three studies listed, and it hails from 18 years ago. It was published in the journal *Birth*. It may interest the reader to know that *Birth* is published on behalf of Lamaze International, just like the *Journal of Perinatal*

---

[1] **Perinatal mortality** means death of the fetus or newborn near the time of birth. It generally includes fetal deaths toward the end of pregnancy, deaths during labor and birth, and deaths that occur during the first week of life.

Education.

Because Olsen's meta-analysis was completed in 1997, all of the six studies included are rather aged (ranging from 1977 to 1994) and four of the six studies are international. International studies are of limited value due to the extreme differences in midwifery training from country to country. The two U.S. studies included, Mehl (1977 in Wisconsin) and Durand (1992 in Tennessee), are not only small (sample sizes equal to or less than 1707) and one could argue outdated, but they also are not included in MANA's list of "best evidence" for home birth safety. If MANA is going to hold up a meta-analysis as best-evidence, why would they not include the studies that powered the meta-analysis on the same list?

Olsen concluded in 1997 that, "No empirical evidence exists to support the view it is less safe for most low-risk women to plan a home birth." It allows the reader to hope that as we move into more recent research, a stronger conclusion (such as evidence supporting that it is safe, rather than a lack of evidence that it isn't) could be reached.

Section II: Randomized Controlled Trials

Hendrix et al: Moving on to section II, labeled Randomized Controlled Trials (RCTs), I am once again wondering how RCTs can be ethically conducted to study birthplace. I quickly realize that in this section only two studies are listed, and the first one, by Hendrix et al, is self-explanatory in its title: "Why women do not accept randomization for place of birth." This paper only indicates that the researchers failed at attempting an RCT.

Dowswell et al: The second (and last) study in this section is by Dowswell. It sounds familiar because it was reviewed by Olsen and Clausen and encompassed only eleven participants. Considering the relative rarity of birth complications, a study with eleven participants is not useful.

Section III: Cohort and Population-Based Observational Studies

Janssen et al 2009: Section III, Cohort and Population-Based Observational Studies, proves to be where the meat is. The first study listed,

"Outcomes of planned home births with registered midwife versus planned hospital birth with midwife or physician" was published in the Canadian Medical Association Journal in 2009. In this study, conducted in British Columbia, Canada, home birth mothers experienced fewer interventions, lower morbidity (sickness or injury), and lower neonatal[2] morbidity and mortality. The perinatal death rate was .35 per 1000, compared to .57-.64 per thousand for hospital-based midwife- and physician-attended births respectively. (At this point, I realize that Gulbranson's New Zealand study, with a perinatal death rate of nearly 3 in one thousand, compares very unfavorably with Janssen's rate, at over eight times higher; I wonder how Leslie and Romano justified including both Janssen's rate and Gulbranson's much higher rate in the same category and calling them "similar" in their systematic review.) The Janssen study is well-designed, featuring totally respectable numbers of women enrolled and fair comparison groups. Before I considered this study a total win for home birth, however, I pressed in on a couple of details.

_____

[2] The **neonatal** period refers to the time after birth and before 28 days of life.

Canadian Registered Midwives
and U.S. Midwives Compared

First, registered midwives in Canada are quite different, in several ways, from the vast majority of home birth midwives in the United States. Registered midwives in Canada have to hold a baccalaureate degree in midwifery. They are trained to give care in both home and the hospital setting. The credential that they could be best compared to in the United States is the Certified Nurse Midwife (CNM). This is the kind of midwife that you usually find working in hospital maternity units, the kind that can prescribe medication and perform many gynecological procedures as well as manage births.

The average home birth midwife in the United States is not a CNM, but what is referred to as a direct-entry midwife (DEM). DEMs attend the vast majority of U.S. nonhospital births. The average DEM is a high school graduate, although that is not technically required. She has gone to school for midwifery, usually for three years if she took a full-time course load. These schools are often distance-learning programs and may or may not be accredited;

if they are accredited, it may be by the state in which they are run or by an organization called MEAC, the Midwifery Education Accreditation Council. The credits earned are not transferrable to state or private universities.

Clinical training for a direct-entry midwife can vary widely. The current standards for an entry-level certified professional midwife indicate that she can begin practicing after having attended as few as 55 births over the course of several years. I attended one of the most clinically rigorous direct-entry midwifery programs in the United States from 2005 to 2008, the International School of Midwifery in Miami, Florida. During my time there I attended over 150 births, 50 of which were my "catches," meaning I was the one who caught the baby as it was born. My clinical training was extensive compared to many direct-entry midwives: I inserted IV's and administered antibiotics, sutured tears, drew blood, inserted catheters, performed pap smears, and many other tasks that many midwives never or rarely do during their training. (Often they lack the opportunity, as such procedures are not permitted in their state.) But as much clinical practice as I got, I was never able to provide care in a hospital setting. Any time I had to bring a client to the hospital, my role changed into that of a support person, not a healthcare provider. Even the most highly trained direct-entry midwife cannot boast that she is truly integrated into the medical care system the way a Canadian registered midwife must be.

Understanding the distinction between a Canadian registered midwife and a DEM from the United States, we now know that we can't draw a direct comparison to home birth in British Columbia (where the midwifery system is completely different) and nonhospital birth in the United States. What other issues are there with this well-done study?

The second is the rigorous exclusion criteria that Canadian registered midwives in British Columbia must adhere to. This includes that the mother must have no significant pre-existing disease, no significant disease arising during pregnancy, a singleton pregnancy (no twins or higher order multiples), the baby must be head-down, labor must start between 37 and 41 weeks of pregnancy, the mother must have had no more than 1 previous caesarean section, and labor must begin spontaneously. These criteria ensure that risk is kept to a minimum, and according to this study it is working up in British Columbia.

The problem I see is that direct entry midwives in the United States will often attend home births that do not fit these criteria; while insisting that home birth is at least as safe as hospital birth, many will attend twin births, breech births, births after 41 weeks, births of women who have pre-existing or pregnancy-induced disease, births after two or more previous caesarean sections, and births of women whose labor has been jump-started rather than begun spontaneously (whether by herbs, prolonged nipple stimulation, the breaking of her water, or illicit use of medications). I doubt I could find a single direct-entry midwife who hasn't attended a birth outside of the parameters that Canadian registered midwives must follow. This means, of course, that the results of this study cannot be extrapolated to the United States as midwifery is currently practiced.

The bottom line of the Janssen study is that home birth with a registered midwife in British Columbia was demonstrated to be at least as safe as hospital birth, provided the strict exclusion criteria was applied. Would I see this trend continue as I moved forward?

Hutton et al: Quite literally, the trend continued, in that the next study was also Canadian: "Outcomes associated with planned home and planned hospital births in low-risk women attended by midwives in Ontario, Canada, 2003-2006," not surprisingly shows similar results to the Janssen study. Published by *Birth* (sponsored by Lamaze International), the Hutton study shows lower rates of interventions such as cesarean section, episiotomy, and medical pain relief for the home birth group. It also shows that the perinatal mortality rate was not significantly different between home and hospital.

It seemed that Canada was an example of a successful home birth system. Two studies have supported that not only were fewer interventions used, but perinatal outcomes were as safe as the hospital. Perhaps in the following studies I would find that the same is true in the United States.

Section III: Cohort/Population Studies (Continued)

Johnson & Daviss: Letter C under section III of the list of studies that the Midwives Alliance of

North America deems the very best in proving home birth safety is titled, "Outcomes of planned home birth with certified professional midwives." Published in the *British Medical Journal* by Johnson and Daviss in 2005, this study promises to finally demonstrate what U.S. direct-entry midwives really provide. The planned home birth outcomes included much lower rates of epidural, episiotomy, and assisted delivery, and cesarean section. None of the mothers in the study died. The perinatal death rate was reported at 1.7 in 1000.

This number seems high. Just a few studies ago in Canada, the home birth perinatal death rate was .35 in 1000 (Janssen 2009). 1.7 in 1000 is *over four times higher.* Yet, the study abstract says that this number is "in line" with other established perinatal death rates. Is that true?

The CDC provides the public with access to linked birth and death records for infants as part of a database project called WONDER (Wide-ranging Online Data for Epidemiologic Research). A major limitation of this database is that it does not include intrapartum[3] deaths, because those babies are not issued birth certificates. Fortunately for me, Johnson and Daviss included a breakdown of how many deaths in their study were intrapartum (5) and how many were neonatal (6), which meant a neonatal death rate of 1.1 per 1000.

Using the WONDER database for the year 2000 (the same year Johnson and Daviss collected their data), I plugged in the following variables: all babies who died within 27 days of birth, born in the hospital, who were at least 37 weeks gestation, with a known attendant type (type of doctor or midwife). I did not exclude any risk factors except prematurity, which should always be screened out as high-risk for home birth. The neonatal death rate was 0.99 per 1000.

This 0.99/1000 hospital neonatal death rate included women with pregnancy complications that would make them too high-risk for even the most experienced (or foolish) midwife to take on. It included the diabetic, pregnant mothers on illicit drugs, the morbidly obese, the poverty-stricken, and those who received no prenatal care at all. It included practically

---

[3] **Intrapartum** refers to the time during the labor and birth process. Intrapartum deaths occur before the birth of the baby.

every mother in the U.S. who made it to full-term and got herself to a hospital, regardless of health, socioeconomic status, or pregnancy complications. It also included lethal congenital anomalies, which were excluded from Johnson and Daviss' numbers. (Including lethal congenital anomalies the Johnson and Daviss neonatal death rate was 1.6/1000.) The neonatal death rate including the depth and breadth of risk at hospital births was *lower* than the self-selected, "low-risk," health-conscious group who tends to choose home birth that Johnson and Daviss studied.

Women who choose nonhospital birth are not a random sample of the overall birthing population; they are self-selected, and (supposedly) carefully screened by their midwives to ensure they are "low risk." The overall mortality rate for all-risk term pregnancies across the board ought to be significantly higher than the mortality rate for the "low-risk" women who decide on nonhospital birth. It seems as if women are trading their low-risk status in for a nonhospital birth, and thereby actually becoming higher in risk than the general population. If nonhospital birth were just as safe for low-risk women, it ought to be beating all-risk

21

hospital birth hands-down in every aspect of safety. If nonhospital birth isn't showing a clear lead, we have a problem.

I also plugged some variables into WONDER to try to approximate the year 2000 hospital neonatal death rate for low-risk women specifically. I tried to match Johnson and Daviss as specifically as possible by adding in the additional variables of singleton (not twins or other multiples) and looking at Certified Nurse Midwives, who tend to care for lower-risk mothers than obstetricians. Their neonatal mortality rate was 0.58, less than half Johnson and Daviss' rate, both groups including congenital anomalies. Some may argue that CNMs' death rates are lowered by the fact that their more complicated cases get referred to obstetricians; that is true. But direct-entry midwives ought to be referring their more complicated cases to obstetricians as well, enjoying the very same benefit. Obstetricians take on all other providers' most complicated cases, at every stage of complication, and they still maintain a lower death rate than Johnson and Daviss demonstrated.

Lies, Damn Lies, and Statistics

I had first heard about these numbers years ago, when I was still practicing, long before that morning with the binder and the coffee. I had read enough to know that giving birth with a direct-entry midwife like myself meant, statistically speaking, an approximate two- to threefold risk of death to the babies I caught compared to the same birth in a hospital setting. A client would sometimes come to me with concerns: "My mother doesn't approve, she says she doesn't think it is safe." "My husband saw something on the news." "I found something on the Internet." I would gently explain to her the logic that allowed me to continue: the difference between relative risk and absolute risk, and the fact that the absolute risk seemed so very small.

"The best statistics show that it might be *slightly* more dangerous for the baby, but your chances of intervention are *much* lower. And three times a very small number is still a very small number," I would say, looking into her eyes earnestly. Sometimes admitting a little weakness can buy a lot of trust. Inevitably, the client would agree with me:

chances were, she would have a lovely birth if she stuck with me. It didn't seem like such a gamble. Chances were, bad things would only happen to someone else, somewhere else, on another day.

As for me, I would put it out of my mind. I focused on giving the best prenatal care I could. I focused on monitoring the baby well during labor and helping moms feel as comfortable as possible. I focused on building moms up and coaching them to hang in there and believe in themselves. And inevitably, when I started to see the baby's head, I felt nothing but relief that we were going to see a baby soon. Equally inevitably, whenever the baby's head reached about the halfway point, at that moment when a new face is about to appear in the world for the first time, I would have a moment of sheer terror deep in my gut: *What are you DOING. This is absurd. This better go well. You better hope this goes well.*

At such moments I often felt as if I had an out-of-body experience, as if I were simply watching myself performing the actions of a midwife, supporting the baby's slippery body as it tumbled out, making sure he started to breathe, getting him warm and dry and cuddled up with mom, and turning my attention to the placenta. I often received accolades from observers who would say I "kept my cool" under every circumstance. Call me Meryl Streep; I know how to play the role of the confident midwife. No one ever knew that deep down I was terrified.

Section III: Cohort/Population Studies (Re-Continued)

Johnson & Daviss Continued: Still considering Johnson and Daviss, I wondered how this study could be considered by MANA to be among the best evidence for the safety of home birth, seeing as it shows a perinatal death rate higher than hospital births from the same time. In their words, "Intrapartum and neonatal death rates were compared with… comparable studies of low risk hospital births." I looked over the list of the ten studies the authors chose, which numbers permitted the authors to conclude that their death rate was "similar" to hospital birth. The most recent study listed was dated 2002, and the name of the researcher was familiar: Janssen, the same author of the 2009 Canadian study I just looked at. Johnson and Daviss were referencing Janssen's earlier study, also conducted in

Canada, wherein the hospital perinatal death rate was 1.36 per thousand, but the sample size was only 733 women and there was exactly one death.

The other studies dated mostly to the 1980s. The oldest included study used data collected from 1969-1975. Johnson and Daviss apparently had to reach back into the 1960s to find low-risk hospital numbers that would make their death rate seem "similar." Perhaps the fact that Daviss is a midwife, and Johnson is her husband and noted midwifery advocate, were motivating factors in the selection of comparison studies.

Janssen et al 2002: Still making my way through the MANA list of best evidence for the safety of home birth, the next study sounds familiar: Janssen et al present, "Outcomes of planned home births versus planned hospital births after regulation of midwifery in British Columbia, 2002." Not surprisingly, this study showed that home birth with a Canadian registered midwife had a lower incidence of almost every kind of obstetric intervention. However, there were a few incidents the authors reported that were not statistically significant due to small sample size, but worth noting: the only two cases of obstetric shock occurred in home births, and three of the four blood transfusions in the study were after home births. Three cases of perinatal death occurred in the home birth group (out of 860 cases), compared to only one death in the hospital group (733 cases). Short case reports were given of all three deaths in the home birth group, suggesting that none of them were likely related to birthplace or attendant. Five babies in the home birth group received assisted ventilation for over 24 hours compared to 0 of the hospital births, a statistically significant finding.

Overall, this study is not as ringing an endorsement of Canadian home birth as the follow up in 2009 (already reviewed) would seem to be. Indeed, in a letter to the publishing journal dated June of 2011, Janssen herself responded to criticisms of this study, writing that "selection bias is unavoidable" when studying home birth, and that her study suffered from a "lack of power" to make "valid conclusions." With such a "recommendation" from the author, it is interesting that MANA has left it in this list of "best evidence."

Schlenzka: That brings me to the final study cited in section III: an unpublished dissertation by

Schlenzka, dated 1999. An unpublished dissertation is a notable departure from the rest of this list. Although one can argue about possible bias in journals that publish research articles, all real research journals subject all articles to at least a cursory (and, in most highly regarded journals, a truly rigorous) peer review, the process by which other experts fact-check the study and ensure that at least a minimum level of trustworthiness and quality is met. An unpublished dissertation, on the other hand, has literally no known standard for accuracy. The author could write falsehoods, misinterpret data, make grievous factual errors, and misquote sources, and there is no system of accountability.

To place an unpublished dissertation alongside published peer-reviewed studies seems naively disingenuous at best and deliberately deceptive at worst. If this dissertation, dated 1999, is some of the best evidence for the safety of home birth, why hasn't it at least been picked up by one of Lamaze International's sponsored journals?

Section IV: International Observational Studies

The next category comprises international cohort and population-based observational studies. This collection of eight studies is of limited use to anyone trying to determine safety of home birth in the United States due to the substantial differences between direct-entry midwifery in the U.S. and the hospital-trained midwives of other countries. I reviewed all of them anyway.

Birthplace in England: The first international study is from England, published in 2011 in the *British Medical Journal*. It determined that women who had given birth previously had outcomes just as good when giving birth at home as in the hospital; however, women having their first baby at home experienced poorer perinatal outcomes (more deaths and injuries).

Van der Kooy et al: The second study, published in 2011, hailed from the Netherlands and determined that Dutch home births are: "under routine conditions… not associated with a higher intrapartum and early neonatal mortality rate. However, in subgroups, additional risk cannot be excluded." I quote the study because quite honestly, having read it, I cannot really figure out what it means about the subgroups. Suffice it to say that they haven't completely ruled out an increase in risk for Dutch home birth, but they did not find an increase in risk.

de Jonge et al: The third study, published in 2009, is also from the Netherlands. De Jonge explains that in the Netherlands about 30% of women plan to give birth at home; the Netherlands also has one of the highest perinatal death rates in Europe. This study found no significant difference in outcomes between planned home and hospital births attended by midwives. (De Jonge did not provide a comparison to hospital births attended by obstetricians. In later reading I discovered that a 2010 study by Evers et al would demonstrate that "low-risk" births attended by Dutch midwives have a higher perinatal death rate than high-risk births attended by Dutch obstetricians, indicating that midwives in the Netherlands have poor statistics regardless of birthplace.)

Kennare et al: The fourth study is from South Australia (2009) and, remarkably, found that although home birth in South Australia carries about the same risk of neonatal death as hospital birth, the risk of intrapartum (during labor) fetal death is seven times that of hospital birth, and the risk of death from intrapartum asphyxia (lack of oxygen) is 27 times higher! Intrapartum asphyxia is a cause of death that ought to be avoidable with proper fetal monitoring. This is included in a list of the best evidence for the safety of home birth?! But this was one rather small study in Australia, so I'll move on.

Chamberlain et al: The next study listed, *Home Births: The Report of the 1994 Confidential Inquiry by the National Birthday Trust Fund*, was conducted in Great Britain and was published in the form of a book in 1997. According to the blurb on Amazon.com, the study "shows that planned birth at home is a safe option, that the women who are being selected for home births are appropriate, and that midwives manage home births well and competently." Due to the outdatedness of the information and the fact that birth with a medically-trained British midwife tells us very little about the safety of home birth with an American direct-entry midwife, I found this study to be irrelevant to my quest to determine the safety of nonhospital birth in the United States.

Ackermann-Liebrich et al: The sixth study is from Switzerland in 1996 and determined that, "The number of participants was too small to detect differences either in maternal or perinatal mortality between the groups."

Wiegers et al: The seventh study is from the Netherlands, published in 1996, and actually does conclude that home birth in the Netherlands is at least as safe as hospital birth. This is the first study to use the phrase, "at least as good," which probably inspired the very common phrase "at least as safe" when talking about nonhospital birth. Unfortunately, a 19-year-old study from a country with a completely different midwifery and health care system tells us nothing about current home birth in the U.S.

Northern Region: The last study in this section is from Great Britain and found no significant difference in risk between home and hospital birth from 1981 to 1994.

The takeaway from this collection of international studies seemed to be that, in the right circumstances, with highly qualified midwives well-integrated into the medical system, home birth can be as safe as hospital birth. However, with half of these studies dating 1996 or 1997, it seems that there should be more up-to-date information available from these countries with successful and safe home birth programs.

Section V: Descriptive Studies

The last section in the MANA list is Section V: Descriptive Studies and Registry Reports Observational Studies: International. Although they are titled "international," only two of these studies are based outside of the U.S., so I hope to get more applicable information here.

MacDorman, Declercq, & Menacker: The first study, published in 2011, seeks to describe women (by race and ethnicity) who plan home births in contrast with women who experience unplanned home births. This study makes neither examination of nor claims as to safety.

Declercq, MacDorman, Menacker, & Stotland: The second study, published in 2010, is an examination of the difference between planned and unplanned home births. The conclusion is that unplanned home births involve many higher risk factors than planned home births, and that states should be tracking those two groups separately.

Although this study has nothing to do with safety outcomes (and therefore perhaps should not be included in this list at all), it does point out something important: birth certificate data does not reveal which births are planned to occur at home but transport to the hospital. This means that safety data encoded into birth certificate paperwork will always attribute some poor outcomes to the hospital when they might more accurately belong to planned home births.

Amelink-Verburg et al: The third study was published in 2008 and is very specific to the Dutch medical system and has to do with categories of referrals within that system. Perhaps the only use for this study outside of the Netherlands is to demonstrate how very different (and truly incomparable) our system is.

Murphy & Fullerton: The fourth study, published in 1998, describes outcomes of home births with Certified Nurse Midwives (CNM) in the United States. A CNM is a nurse with a master's degree in nurse-midwifery. This study showed a perinatal mortality rate of 2.5 per 1000, a rate that strikes me as incredibly high. (Remember, the Canadian perinatal mortality rate in the Janssen study was .35

34

per thousand.) However, since this study came out in 1998, I admit that I don't have a readily available comparison group, and the study does not provide one. The study itself cites two studies from the mid-1980s with lower perinatal mortality rates in uncomplicated hospital birth. Also, this study had a small sample size of 1404. Overall, my impression is that home birth with a CNM in the U.S. needs an updated and more detailed study to draw conclusions.

Cawthon: The fifth study was created by and submitted to the state of Washington in 1996. It compared women on Medicaid who had home births with Medicaid women who had hospital births. This study shows that although women who receive care from a licensed midwife in Washington State experienced low rates of perinatal death when delivering at home, the women who received care from a midwife but had to transport to the hospital for birth experienced a very high perinatal death rate of nearly 3%. This probably indicates that licensed midwives often transport in time for the hospital to be stuck with the poor outcome, but too late for the baby to be saved. The same study looked at Certified Nurse Midwives and found no significant difference in outcomes between the Medicaid births they attended at home and Medicaid births in the hospital.

Anderson & Murphy: This brings me to the very last study on MANA's list of the "best" evidence for the safety of home birth. This 1995 study (by the same Murphy from the 1998 study listed above) is a look at outcomes of births attended by Certified Nurse Midwives from 1987-1991. The perinatal mortality rate in this study was found to be two per thousand, slightly lower than the 2.5 per thousand that would be found by Murphy in her follow-up study three years later (reviewed above). This rate, while substantially higher than the .35 per thousand benchmark from the Janssen study, must be viewed in light of the fact that the data is quite dated.

The hours I had spent combing over all of MANA's best evidence led me to this conclusion: nonhospital birth might be as safe as hospital birth, but likely only in health systems in which midwives are hospital-trained and well-integrated, and where exclusion criteria are strictly observed to permit only the lowest risk women to proceed. Nonhospital birth in the United States as currently practiced is responsible for lower numbers of interventions (such as cesarean section and medical pain relief) but a substantially higher risk of death or injury to the baby.

Unbelievably, our "own" evidence, upon close inspection, was almost unanimously against us. But I wasn't quite finished with MANA-related data, because there was one study not on the list that originated from MANA itself.

The MANA Study

Cheney et al: In 2014, Cheney et al published "Outcomes of Care for 16,924 Planned Home Births in the United States: The Midwives Alliance of North America Statistics Project, 2004-2009" (AKA "the MANA study") in the *Journal of Midwifery and Women's Health*, the official journal of the American College of Nurse-Midwives. A notable strength of this study was that it tracked planned home births regardless of where the women ended up giving birth, information that is impossible to gather from birth certificate data. A substantial majority (at least 13,400 of 16,924) of the home births (birth center births were excluded from the study) were attended by direct-entry midwives; an additional 2613 were attended by

CNM midwives (or the similarly-trained, hospital-credentialed Certified Midwives), and the remainder were attended by attendants that do not fit either category, such as students, naturopathic doctors, and chiropractors.

The study revealed that planned home birth results in a low Caesarean rate of 5.3% (compared to the 32.7% nationwide average reported by the CDC in 2013) and a very high breastfeeding initiation rate of over 99% (compared to the overall nationwide rate of 79.2%). Maternal outcomes included one death.

The intrapartum (during-labor) fetal death rate in the MANA study was reported at 1.3 per 1000. It is difficult to find a comparison rate for this number, as the stillbirth statistics in the general population include babies who are not yet full-term as well as full-term babies who die before the onset of labor. Of course, we still have the Janssen study from Canada, which provided us with a comparison rate of .35 per thousand perinatal (during-labor plus neonatal) deaths. Using the Janssen study as a standard, we can see that MANA loses over three times as many babies during labor as Canada loses during labor and the neonatal period combined.

The early neonatal death rate (death after birth but before seven days of life) on the other hand is fairly simple to compare with other rates. The MANA neonatal death rate was 1.29 per 1000. I used the WONDER database to again try to ascertain a comparison group. Using the same years as the MANA study, 2004-2009, I included all term hospital births with a known attendant type that died within 27 days. (I had to average two databases in order to encompass those years.) The hospital neonatal death rate for births with those criteria was .85 per thousand. The low-risk MANA home birth neonatal death rate is over 50% higher. This is especially stunning considering the depth and breadth of complicated cases included in the hospital numbers. MANA's "low-risk" population should be beating the general population hands-down when it comes to newborn survival, if home birth is indeed as safe as hospital birth.

The Other Side

The next step seemed to be to look at what literature MANA had neither generated nor opted to include in their list of "best evidence." MANA had not provided me with a handy list of opposing information, so I needed to search it out myself.

Grunebaum et al 2013: The *American Journal of Obstetrics & Gynecology* addressed choice of birthplace twice in October of 2013. The first, "Apgar score of 0 at 5 minutes and neonatal seizures or serious neurologic dysfunction in relation to birth setting," by Grunebaum et al, examined birth setting by the outcome of a zero Apgar at five minutes. The Apgar score is assigned to every baby at one and five minutes of life, regardless of birthplace, as long as the attendant is trained to assign one. The score is reported on birth certificate data. A "perfect" score of ten indicates a baby that is vigorous, well-oxygenated, and transitioning very well to extrauterine life. A baby with an Apgar score of 0 at five minutes essentially means the baby had no signs of life at that time; a baby with no signs of life at 5 minutes of age may or may not survive, and if they do they will likely suffer from severe brain damage. This study found that babies had 3.56 times the risk of Apgar 0 at 5 minutes when born with midwives at a birth center, and 10.55 times the risk when born with midwives at home.

Nonhospital births also carried significantly higher risk of neonatal seizure or serious neurologic dysfunction.

It is important to address the fact that the use of birth certificate data is not perfect. First of all, although hospital births always include the filing of birth certificate data, the same cannot be said of all home births. Especially in states where midwifery is illegal, midwives do not always fill out or submit birth certificate data. The parents will often submit the birth certificate paperwork themselves, and may or may not submit an Apgar score with any accuracy. Secondly, when a woman is transported to the hospital during labor because something isn't going right at a planned nonhospital birth, the hospital has no way of indicating on the birth certificate data that the birth was an aborted home birth attempt. Therefore, the data on hospital deaths includes most homebirth transfers that ended in tragedy. Those babies are recorded as hospital deaths or grave injuries and not as nonhospital deaths or grave injuries. Thus, it is not only likely, but assuredly the case, that these numbers for neonatal mortality are underestimating the number of deaths and injuries to babies that can be attributed to planned nonhospital birth, perhaps drastically.

Cheng et al: In the same issue of *AJOG*, Cheng et al published an analysis of the CDC data that focused on low 5-minute Apgar scores at two thresholds, below four and below seven, as well as neonatal seizure. Cheng found that babies born at home had a nearly two-fold increased chance of a five-minute Apgar below four, and over twice the chance of a five-minute Apgar below seven. Cheng also found that the chance of neonatal seizure was over three times higher in the home birth group. Cheng reported that women who give birth at home are much less likely to experience obstetric interventions such as antibiotic use, induction of labor, and the use of vacuum or forceps-assisted delivery. The paper concluded that planned home births resulted in a trade-off, with fewer obstetric interventions received but a significantly increased chance of neonatal complications.

Grunebaum et al 2014: In January 2014, Grunebaum et al took another look at birthplace safety and published an analysis of CDC data not unlike the informal one I did for this paper. They found that hospital midwives had a neonatal death rate of

.31/1000, a number strikingly similar to Janssen's Canadian homebirth numbers discussed earlier. Midwives working in a nonhospital birth center had a neonatal death rate of .63/1000, double the rate of death compared to the hospital, and home birth midwives had a neonatal death rate of 1.32/1000, over four times the risk of neonatal death compared to the hospital midwives. Grunebaum's findings can be further expressed by explaining that for every 10,000 babies born at home with a midwife, about ten will die a death that would have been preventable in the hospital.

Rooks: With this literature arising from the obstetric world, the reader may wonder if any midwives had noticed a similar trend. I was able to find one who had: in 2013 a Certified Nurse Midwife in Oregon named Judith Rooks not only identified the trend, but submitted a report to the state legislature detailing her findings. She found that nonhospital births with direct-entry midwives in Oregon carried six to eight times the risk of perinatal death compared to hospital births. She ended her letter to the Oregon legislature in a poignant fashion: "In 2012 six Oregon mothers lost their babies in births attended by DEMs.

They may feel guilty about having chosen a home birth with a DEM and are unlikely to lobby their legislators. The more than a thousand women who had good outcomes and are happy are the ones who will call you… Please keep the six women who lost their babies last year in mind as you legislate this year."

My Days as a Midwife Close

Judith Rooks' words seem especially prescient from where I sit in South Carolina, where three babies have recently died after being born at the birth center I started. By 2012, my belief that I was doing good for the world as a midwife had seriously waned. I was haunted by the knowledge that, statistically speaking, we were putting lives at risk with every baby we caught. I was frustrated by disagreements with my partners over issues of safety. Yet, I was not yet willing to walk away from my life's work, my successful business, my social support network, and my position of prestige as a health care provider.

As a distraction, I latched on to issues that soothed my ego, such as achieving better racial diversity in midwifery. The stress of my mental unease wore on me. I picked fights with my partners when they would not stand with me on the racial diversity issue, and years of tension culminated in them kicking me out of the business that I had started. They gave me ten minutes to gather my things and leave the building. As I drove home, I gripped the steering wheel tightly, my heart racing in my chest. *I GOT OUT.* It was messy and confusing and ugly, but I was out of there for good. I was relieved, but I wasn't ready to be honest with the world about why.

That was January 2013. In April 2013, I heard the first rumors of a baby's death soon after her birth at the center. In September 2013, news of a second death was splashed across local newspapers. And in January 2015, a third death was reported. My thoughts and emotions ran rampant. One moment, I would arrogantly congratulate myself: *No deaths on my watch, and three on theirs, who's the best midwife now?* Another moment, I would wonder at my favored status in the universe, that God had spared me from all the horror, and just in time. And in my most honest moments, I knew the truth of it: I had gotten incredibly, ridiculously lucky. And those three mothers who sat at home with empty arms, they simply had not.

As I perused the comments section of the news articles online, a common rejoinder from midwives and their supporters stood out again and again: "But, babies die in hospitals all the time, and that doesn't make the news!" A mistaken response indeed, as the death of full-term, otherwise healthy infants of low-risk mothers in the hospital is vanishingly rare; the vast majority of babies who die in the hospital are premature, have severe anomalies, or are born to high-risk mothers. The birth center experienced three deaths of full-term infants, born to (supposedly) low-risk mothers, all before the center had a chance to reach the 1000-birth benchmark; based on rumors in the blogosphere, the center was closing in on 700 births total. The birth center in Fort Mill closed its doors on the last day of February, 2015.

By the first week of January, 2013, my stint as a licensed midwife was wrapping up, even though I didn't know it at the time. The same mother with the straight blond hair lay in front of me, about to deliver her second child with me in the very same room where she had safely delivered her first a few years before. She was calm; she knew this was "as safe as life gets." I felt the relief at the long-awaited sighting of the top of her baby's head; I felt that predictable, well-hidden panic in my chest as forehead gave way to face and head and shoulders tumbled out; I felt that tight wad of anxiety release as that baby mustered up a lusty cry. I waited watchfully for the placenta, delivering it carefully into a bowl, and massaged the mother's uterus thoroughly to prevent excessive bleeding. I breathed. Once again, I had made it through without disaster. This would not be my one in a thousand. My one in a thousand would never come. Bad things would only happen to someone else, somewhere else, on another day.

A few years removed from the active practice of midwifery now, I find myself wondering how I allowed myself to become so convinced that having and encouraging others to have a nonhospital birth was such a good idea. I called up a friend who had two home births, the last one with me, and asked her, "If you had to buy a car seat for your baby, and one car seat had been rated by Consumer Reports as having two to three times the risk of death or profound injury compared to other car seats, would you buy that car seat?" "Of course not," she replied. "What if it was the most beautiful, comfortable car seat in the world, really easy to carry around, easy to install, and your baby would just love sitting in it?" I continued. "No way," she replied. "What would you say about a parent who did buy that car seat?" I asked. "I'd say they were making a poor decision."

Why?

In my new life as a student of psychology, I want to understand why people make the decisions that they do. The research is clear that nonhospital birth with a midwife reduces obstetric interventions but substantially increases risk of death and profound injury to babies. MANA's own hand-picked data bears witness to an increased risk by a factor of at least two or three, as does MANA's own study. The obstetric data is even more unforgiving, showing risk of death at nonhospital birth between four and ten times that of the hospital. So, why is it that thousands of intelligent, well-educated, and economically advantaged women are choosing nonhospital birth every year? Is it because they don't know the facts? Or is it because they feel that a dramatically higher chance of death or injury to their newborn is not as important a consideration as their desire for fewer obstetric interventions?

Original Survey Research

In the winter of 2015 I conducted an online survey of 1,057 women regarding their experiences, attitudes, and beliefs regarding nonhospital births. These women were recruited via Facebook, including in groups that targeted women interested in the topic of natural birth. Ages ranged from 19 to 71, with a mean age of 34 years old. At least 447 nonhospital births were planned. At least 1,456 births to the participants occurred in a hospital setting. Any uncounted births are due to participants selecting the "four or more" options for each category. 56 of the planned nonhospital births transported to the hospital during labor and are counted in both groups.

Of the participants who had hospital births, the most popular reasons for choosing the hospital included feeling like it was the safest place for the mom and baby, the fact that it was covered by insurance, and a desire for access to medical interventions. Among participants who chose nonhospital birth, the top reasons included a desire to avoid interventions, wanting more comfortable surroundings, a belief that birth does not require hospitalization, and the feeling that nonhospital birth was the safest choice.

53% of women who chose nonhospital birth indicated that they had consulted scientific journals when making their decision, compared with only 33% of hospital birthers. The women who chose nonhospital consulted most with a midwife, followed closely by their spouse or partner. The women who chose hospital birth consulted most with their spouse or partner, followed by a doctor.

I found that 87% of women who planned nonhospital birth agreed with the statement, "Generally speaking, giving birth in a non-hospital setting is at least as safe as giving birth in a hospital for low-risk women" (69% strongly agreed). One might suppose that experiencing complications at a nonhospital birth might change women's perspectives, but I did not find this to be the case. I isolated the 74 women who had experienced transport (i.e., they or their baby were taken to the hospital during labor or shortly after birth) into a subgroup and found that 81% agreed with the "at least as safe" statement (and 64% strongly agreed). By contrast, only 43% of women who had never planned a nonhospital birth agreed that nonhospital birth was "at least as safe."

When asked about the statement, "Having a safe and healthy mother and baby are the only things that truly matter in birth," 68% of the women who had only had hospital births agreed with this statement. Of the women who planned nonhospital birth, only 36% agreed with this statement, and 50% disagreed (remainder neutral).

Women who choose nonhospital birth are overwhelmingly satisfied with their experience. Of the women who planned a nonhospital birth, 78.7% reported being "Very Satisfied" with their first nonhospital birth experience, increasing to 87.9% at the second nonhospital birth. By contrast, only 38.8% of the participants were "very satisfied" with their first hospital birth experience. In addition, women who plan a nonhospital birth are highly likely to recommend nonhospital birth to other women, with 59% reporting they would "definitely" recommend it and an additional 20% reporting they would "probably" recommend nonhospital birth.

Justification

Why are women so overwhelmingly satisfied with nonhospital birth? It is likely that the answer lies in the unavailability of effective pain control. This may sound ridiculous on its face: how could a more painful experience lead to higher satisfaction rates? But as Elliot Aronson and Carol Tavris explain in their book *Mistakes Were Made (But Not By Me),* "…if people go through a great deal of pain, discomfort, effort, or embarrassment to get something, they will be happier with that 'something' than if it came to them easily." Dr. Aronson found that when students are put through a more severe hazing process, they are much more satisfied with the resulting club membership than students who are put through a relatively mild initiation procedure. It follows that women who choose to experience more pain, discomfort, or effort during childbirth would be more satisfied with their birth than women who did not choose that experience. Speaking for myself, I remember being totally thrilled with my first birth, even though it was one of the most physically painful experiences of my life. But why are we more satisfied after experiencing more pain?

People with good self-esteem tend to view themselves in a positive way. I like to think of myself as competent, knowledgeable, educated, sensible, and a maker of good decisions. Therefore, when we make decisions that cause ourselves pain, we are psychologically driven to justify it. "I am a smart person who makes good decisions" and "I just chose to put myself through a lot of pain" are two thoughts that, when entertained in the mind at the same time, produce an uncomfortable state known as "cognitive dissonance." When we experience cognitive dissonance, our minds immediately find justifications: "It was worth it because..." and we fill in the blanks. It was worth it because I love my baby more for it; it was worth it because my baby is healthier for it, which means I'm a better mother; it was worth it because I didn't have to have any interventions; it was worth it because now I know I can do anything! My brain distorts my perceptions of the event so that I see only the upsides, and ignore any downsides. The result? I can maintain my sense of self: I'm a smart person who makes good decisions, and if I chose pain, it must have been for very smart and good reasons.

For most of human history, pain in childbirth was almost unavoidable for women. Indeed, in many parts of the world today, women have no choice as to whether they feel the pain of labor and birth. For women without a choice, there is no experience of cognitive dissonance; they have no need to justify their pain. It is only among women who have access to effective pain relief yet choose to forego it that self-justification becomes activated. They are not going through pain in order to get a baby, because they could opt for pharmaceutical pain relief if they so chose and still get a baby out of the deal, as so many of their acquaintances surely have done. They are opting to experience the pain so that they can achieve a natural, drug-free birth. As Tavris and Aronson explain, "...if a person voluntarily goes through a difficult or painful experience in order to attain some goal or object, that goal or object becomes more attractive." The fact that women make a free choice to experience the pain of childbirth makes the attainment of a drug-free birth seem like a most worthwhile goal.

Of course, this is not a conscious process.

Women do not believe the pain of birth leads to their view of drug-free birth as a worthy goal; they believe that they loved the experience based on its intrinsic merits. The students who went through the severe hazing process in order to get into a club did not believe that the hazing had anything to do with their enjoyment of the club. Even after a debriefing process in which the entire experiment was explained, they still insisted that they liked the club based on its own merits. The club was designed to be dull and worthless, and students who went though a mild initiation process invariably agreed that it was. It is entirely predictable that women who have chosen a drug-free birth would disagree strongly with the suggestion that the pain of childbirth was a hazing-like process that strongly influenced their estimation of drug-free birth as a wonderful experience.

When self-justification kicks in regarding a choice we have made, people often are driven to proselytize their decision. We feel even better about our choices, and far less dissonant, if we can convince others to make the same decision themselves. Nothing reduces dissonance more than seeing others follow your example: "What a fine example of a person I must be, that others have followed in my footsteps." No wonder women who have experienced a natural, drug-free birth are such big advocates of the practice! Having justified the painful initiation for themselves, they turn to convincing others to choose the same.

Our judgments of others who make different decisions are also a function of self-justification. When a woman chooses not to have a drug-free birth experience, women who believe in the superiority of natural birth tend to think of her as less-than: she took the easy way out; she just doesn't get it; she probably doesn't really care about her health, or her baby's health, as much as I care about mine. We justify our own choices by putting down others'. If we were truly to acknowledge her decision as a perfectly excellent one, it would diminish the stellar quality of our own choice.

The Confirmation Bias

When I was pregnant the first time, I was convinced by many natural birth advocates that giving birth without drugs (and specifically pain medication) was the best possible way to give birth. I met such women in real life, read books written by such, and looked at websites maintained by these advocates. Once I had actually experienced a natural birth, I became one of them. From that point on, my mind only operated in one direction: anything I read that confirmed what I thought and felt about birth, I held up to myself and others as a fine example of logical thinking and scientific understanding. Anything that would argue otherwise, I dismissed as full of errors and bias. These mental gymnastics are not unique to me: they are known as the "confirmation bias," and most people share this tendency. When women wish to research nonhospital birth, they are likely to seek out information that confirms what they wish to believe, regardless of the scientific veracity of the source. They are likely to disregard or avoid information that conflicts with their position, dismissing it as unreliable regardless of its value.

The confirmation bias is also responsible for the fact that we see a lack of evidence against our position as equivalent to evidence in favor of our position. I am reminded of Olsen's conclusion in her meta-analysis: "No empirical evidence exists to support the view it is less safe for most low-risk women to plan a home birth." Those with confirmation bias in favor of home birth read this statement and think that it is strong evidence in their favor; after all, if there was evidence that home birth was unsafe, surely someone would have figured that out by 1997 when Olsen was honestly searching for this evidence! Anyone biased against home birth might simply dismiss Olsen's quote out of hand. Those without bias read this as a neutral statement about a lack of evidence. It speaks to the confirmation bias within MANA that Olsen's conclusion forms a prominent piece of what they present to the public as part of their "best evidence" for the safety of home birth.

Confirmation bias is so powerful, psychologists have noted that when people who already have their minds made up about a topic, exposing them to evidence to the contrary only serves to reinforce their original position. This is why a "true believer" in the safety of nonhospital birth, when confronted with the evidence in this paper, is more likely to believe more intensely than ever that the research is wrong, and that nonhospital birth is safe. Perhaps she will grudgingly concede that the evidence is against her, but this will not stop her from deciding that nonhospital birth was the best decision she could have made. "It was the best decision for *me* and *my* family," she may say. I have heard it many times; I have even said it myself.

Sometimes the facts are unavoidable, and the confirmation bias leads us to find new ways to justify maintaining beliefs. One participant in my survey stated, "[Attempts to discourage women from having a nonhospital birth] generally can be traced to... obsession with infant mortality as the only relevant statistic." How I remember feeling this way when I first stumbled upon the neonatal mortality statistics! Surely a few newborn deaths are "worth it" to avoid hundreds of c-sections? Don't women die from unnecessary c-sections too? When I looked into this, I could find no evidence of an increased rate of maternal death due to unneeded c-sections. More women die after c-sections than after vaginal birth, but they tend to have significant comorbidities (other factors of poor health) that contribute both to the need for c-section and the death.

Indeed, "obsession" with infant mortality as the "only" relevant statistic is a charge that many midwives who actually do know the facts may lay at the feet of anyone who claims that nonhospital birth is an unsafe practice. If avoiding obstetric interventions is incredibly important to an individual mother, such as the survey participant who voiced this opinion, she may choose a nonhospital birth even if she understands the increase in risk to her baby. In my experience, most women do not choose their safety over their baby's safety; most women who choose nonhospital birth think they are making a choice that is safer for both herself and her child. They deserve to make a choice based on all the best evidence.

If a mother was considering a nonhospital birth to avoid interventions, even though she was totally aware of the increased risk to her baby, I would encourage her to speak to mothers who have lost babies before making such a choice. I spoke to one such mother online under the condition of anonymity: "I didn't realize the risks when I was pregnant. I thought having a c-section was the worst possible outcome, so I chose home birth to avoid that. I wish to God I hadn't abhorred the idea of a c-section so much. I lost my child because I chose home birth, and I wouldn't have at the hospital. I wish I would have instead been in the hospital, upset that I had a cesarean but holding a live baby, instead of at home with empty arms." I asked her, "How many surgeries is a baby worth?" She replied instantly: "A million."

More Justification

Self-justification kicks into overdrive when we have made an important decision, especially when that decision is irrevocable. As Tavris and Aronson state, "The more costly a decision, in terms of time, money, effort, or inconvenience, and the more irrevocable its consequences, the greater the dissonance and the greater the need to reduce it by overemphasizing the good things about the choice made." To illustrate, the authors describe a study in which bettors at a racetrack were asked how sure they were about their bet both before and after the bet was placed. Gamblers were much more sure they had chosen well once the bet was placed; the choice was made, and the decision irrevocable, so the self-assurance they had made a good choice was much stronger. It is hard to imagine a decision more important or irrevocable than one involving the place and attendant of your child's birth. Therefore, people who have made the decision to have a nonhospital birth and followed through on the birth are especially convinced that it was a smart thing to do. They are unlikely to waver in this conviction, and likely to recommend the practice in glowing terms to others.

The "pyramid of choice," as described in *Mistakes Were Made*, is a phenomenon that can be used to illustrate how people become polarized on the subject of nonhospital birth. Imagine two women standing at the top of a pyramid. They are both deciding whether to plan a hospital birth or a nonhospital birth. There may be very little actual difference between these two women. They could even be identical twins, raised together in the same community, as alike as any two people could be. One decides to give birth at home; the other chooses the hospital. As soon as that choice is made, they move several feet in opposite directions down the pyramid. The one who has chosen hospital birth feels that she has made the best decision for herself, and the one who has chosen home birth feels that she has done likewise. They both seek out friends and writings that support the choices they have made, and move slowly down their respective sides of the pyramid, each becoming more certain through the power of confirmation bias that her choice was the right one. Once the birth has taken place, if all goes well according to the views of that mother, both will have moved all the way down the pyramid to their respective sides. Two women who were previously only a hair's breadth apart now have an entire mountain of difference between them regarding how they view birth.

Self-justification can occur in a chain-like pattern that leads us further and further down the pyramid. When, as a student midwife, I first participated in nonhospital births, I witnessed some things that made me uncomfortable. At my school, the head midwife would sometimes do illegal vacuum-assisted deliveries. The first time I saw one done I didn't realize it was illegal, but when I started talking about it freely, I was quickly quieted by the more senior students. "We call it 'the fruit,'" they said, a reference to the vacuum's brand name, Kiwi. I rationalized that these other students and midwives would not be using "the fruit" if it was really harmful, so the law must be an unnecessary one. Soon, I was recruited to help usher family members out of the room "so the mother can rest," as a cover for the vacuum use; I would then lock the door and stand guard. If I was instructed to cover the mother's face with a cold washcloth "to help her relax," I made sure her eyes were covered so not even she could see the vacuum being applied. I rationalized that surely she would have given us permission to do this to help her get her baby out without transporting, but that it wasn't smart to ask permission to perform an illegal procedure. Toward the end of my apprenticeship, I was the one holding the vacuum, applying it to the baby's head, exerting the carefully angled pressure to help pull the baby down. I rationalized that now I would know how to get a baby out, if I were ever in a situation where there were no available hospitals.

I did not originally plan to attend a school where I would learn to perform dangerous, illegal procedures; I became complicit through a chain reaction of participation and justification. "The fruit" was only one of many "exceptions" I learned to make; many of these exceptions I carried with me to my later practice. Illicit use of medications, cavalier usage of toxic herbs, induction techniques, pretending not to see a cesarean scar, fudging dates, doctoring charts, "accidental" breech deliveries, cheating blood pressure readings, lying to doctors, ignoring borderline test results, pretending to know answers while furtively Googling, waiting just a little bit longer for baby's heart tones to improve, purposely underestimating the staining of amniotic fluid, misrepresenting our personal statistics and the statistical realities of our "profession"… all of these practices are endemic to direct-entry midwifery in the United States. I know because I did most of them. I was present (and silent) as others did them. I heard the stories in "peer review." Not every midwife does all of them; very, very few, if any, do none. It all starts with one small step, and we justify along the way, until we are lost in the woods with no moral compass left to guide us.

Money Talks

The world of direct-entry midwifery suffers from a significant "funding bias," a term that describes people's propensity to emphasize positives and downplay misgivings about the entity that is providing them with money. Midwives make 100% of their income from women who decide to give birth in a nonhospital setting; they are obviously motivated to do everything possible to convince as many people as they can that this is an excellent idea. Midwives at a busy birth center may hit or surpass the six-figure mark during a good year. It is not uncommon for a midwife to earn $2000 or more per birth (after expenses), and some midwives take on 5-6 births on a monthly basis; birth center owners may also take dividends from the business' profits. My take-home pay during our most profitable year would put many obstetricians to shame, and midwives have no student loans to pay off because our educations are dirt-cheap. (My entire midwifery education ran me $3000 in tuition, and this is not unusual.)

Midwives often accuse doctors of being motivated by money, but midwives are at least as motivated by finances as doctors are. Obstetricians in this country are in demand and not likely missing out on much business from the less than two percent of women seeking nonhospital birth; they don't have a financial need to convince women to use the hospital. Midwives on the other hand must drum up interest in natural birth and fear of the hospital in order to keep the dollars rolling in. The thing about bias is, people are unaware of it and defensive toward the suggestion. Midwives' funding bias is something they will never likely examine because no one believes herself to be influenced by money. It is up to the consumer to acknowledge it.

I, the Exception

Both mothers and midwives are guilty of falling under the spell of the "personal fable," a term that refers to a person's perception of herself as unique and special. People tend to think of themselves as the central player in the world, the heroes of their own life stories. Often associated with adolescence, this concept plays into the familiar "invulnerability" attitude that young people are particularly known for. No doubt the, "it might happen to some people, but it won't happen to me" thought process must figure prominently in the minds of women who select a birth scenario with a higher chance of ending in tragedy. (It certainly did in mine.) If a woman knew in advance she would definitely experience a rare but serious complication during birth, it would be a most unusual woman indeed who would want to be far from a modern hospital. The denial that such a complication will occur simply due to its rarity is familiar to most who engage in risky activities.

Midwives also experience a personal fable when they imagine that their actions will never cause harm or death to anyone. If anything goes wrong, it is not our heroine's fault; it must have been bad luck, some dramatic adversity. Thus, whenever a midwife is held accountable for a death or injury that occurred under her purview, it is labeled a "witch-hunt," and dismissed as the work of vindictive obstetricians and overzealous law enforcement. The community rallies around her, showering her with attention and adoration, and often money for her legal defense team.

The Way I Remember It

People tend to think of their own memory as a video recording in their minds that they can rewind and consult at will. Memory doesn't actually work like that, though: as Tavris and Aronson explain, memory is more like a personal historian, who records events in accordance with the perspective and self-concept of the person in question. Memory tends to be a bit of a sycophant; the original spin-doctor, our minds tend to remember us as a little better than we were. Memory tends to forget things that we have done that would be unpleasant, unflattering, or uncomfortable to remember.

During a long, slow labor, I would often wonder why I had chosen a profession that was so dull so much of the time. Obstetricians have notably said that their profession is 99% boredom and 1% sheer terror, and I would have to say that sounds about right to me, at least during the labor part. By the same token, a laboring mother often wonders to herself why having a baby (or having yet another baby) ever seemed like a very good idea in the first place. Memory kindly allows the mother to forget much of the agony of birth, allowing her to consider another baby in the future. Similarly, memory permits the midwife to remember the joy and excitement of catching a baby, and forget the tedium of helping a woman through the labor process, as well as the worry as to whether the baby and mother will make it through the process without significant complication. It seems that this function of memory is adaptive, allowing mothers and midwives to proceed with their business without calling it quits despite the downsides. However, there is a dark side to the revisionist nature of memory in birth.

Women who experience difficult labors, problems, and even serious complications during nonhospital birth often experience cognitive dissonance when they remember and recount the event. The conviction that "I am an intelligent woman who makes good decisions" is dissonant with the fact that she just had a very unpleasant, dangerous, or life-threatening experience at her nonhospital birth. Memory comes to the rescue, and everything gets recast in a light that allows her to continue to see herself (and her midwife, whom she deemed qualified and hired) in a positive way: The labor wasn't that difficult, after all. The problems, they weren't bad, my midwife handled everything well, and it was nothing compared to what could have happened in the hospital. The severe complications could have happened anywhere, to anyone. We can't control everything in life. Besides, my midwife knew exactly when to call 911! And thus, history is re-written. The mother isn't lying when she tells her story. Her own memory has re-written the story to preserve her self-image.

This is how the rampant practice of midwives missing births, which are then attended by whichever unqualified person is closest at hand, continues. A woman pays a nonrefundable amount for a midwife's services, the midwife does not make it in time, and somehow this is generally shared as an amazing story of triumph or a humorous account. It is true that some births are precipitous (very fast), but this problem exceeds the incidence of precipitous labor. How does a midwife maintain a good reputation in the face of missing many births? She flatters the mother: *Wow, you are so amazing, to have done this so fast! You didn't need me at all! Your body knew just what to do.* The mother eagerly internalizes this flattery and remembers that the midwife's absence wasn't really a problem, after all; in fact, it was all part of an exciting, memorable story. She won't hesitate to recommend this midwife to her friends.

Similarly, midwives elude taking responsibility for anything that goes wrong at a birth through their own revision of history. Regardless of how a birth goes, the midwife will remember that she did everything right. If she made a mistake, it was a minor one, perhaps a funny story to tell later. She certainly never put anyone in harm's way. In this way, midwives come to truly believe that they are entirely blameless for anything that goes wrong at a birth. Your midwife isn't lying when she says she's never had any bad outcomes. She believes it to be true. She remembers that any bad outcomes were entirely out of her control, entirely someone else's fault, or no one's fault at all… and therefore, there is no need to disclose that poor outcome to clients. She may also remember many complications as not as bad as they were. Oh, sure, things may have seemed dicey for a while there… but everyone turned out ok in the long run.

I am certainly guilty of allowing my memory to lead me down a primrose path. My memory lingers over moments when I was heroic, times when I saved the day, and events that make me seem, in my own mind, like a smart and responsible caregiver. I have to force myself to see things differently, and it is uncomfortable. That time when I expertly resuscitated that breathless baby? I didn't know he was in distress until he was born; I had missed any warning signs of that. The time I successfully helped a mom avoid the hospital when her blood pressure was a bit high? Her blood pressure was actually dangerously high, and that stunt could have ended in a double tragedy. The time I had to hoist that mom out of the pool and get her on the bed to free her baby's shoulders? (What a hero I was!) Except, she shouldn't have been in that pool at all; she trusted me that it was a good idea to get in there in the first place. And it was only luck that her baby's shoulders freed in time. My memory wants to remember me a certain way, and it is up to me to strive for a more honest perspective.

Me, Accountable?

The peer review process after a midwife presides over a complicated birth is a disturbing procedure. Midwives rarely ask hard questions, such as whether this mother truly was a low-risk candidate, whether or not the midwife was monitoring the baby carefully, and why she decided not to call for help sooner. Most peer review processes are characterized instead by soothing platitudes, an atmosphere of comfort and understanding toward the midwife, and reassuring all participants that they are indeed wonderful, special people.

I will never forget the first truly horrifying hemorrhage I presided over. She was a gorgeous young mother, the very picture of health itself. Her husband was devoted and loving. They were both so eager to have their first baby together at home. The baby came out without much fuss after a couple hours of pushing, but almost as soon as the birth took place, this young mom started bleeding in such copious amounts that it gushingly overcame several of the very large pads we had spread out on her floor. It was a terrifying day that ended with her safe in the hospital, and I was haunted by the memory for months to come.

It was a couple weeks before I had an opportunity to discuss the case at my very first official peer review. A new midwife at the time, I was very eager to hear my fellow midwives' opinions on what I could do differently next time to avoid ever seeing a hemorrhage like that again. I got an answer I was not really looking for: "We know you didn't do anything wrong. *We know you.* We know you're a good midwife. Sometimes things just happen." At the time, it felt flattering, but insincere: they didn't actually know me. They had never attended a birth with me and had spent precious little time with me. They claimed to know me, but what they really knew was what they would want to hear if they were in the hot seat. Peer review was more like an enabling therapeutic back-patting than any form of accountability.

I learned how to play this game, even though it never felt right. You failed to risk someone out? *Well, the birth went well anyway, so your intuition must have been right-on!* You didn't call the second midwife in time for the birth, ten times in a row? *Your mamas sure go fast!* Your client ended up in the hospital needing a blood transfusion? *These things happen in hospitals all the time!* Sometimes I would forget my place and offer a piece of harsh criticism; I was never the most diplomatic person, after all. But this was met with resounding censure: we are here to be *supportive.* I would apologize and get back in line. I felt I had too much to lose to stop playing their game.

The Hurdle to Overcome

When a person does something that is inconsistent with some important aspect of her self-concept, the dissonance is especially painful. Mothers tend to be very invested in themselves as loving and nurturing toward their children; the idea that they put their own children in harm's way creates great dissonance. Midwives, likewise, think of themselves as loving, nurturing, and empowering of women. They enjoy a position of admiration and even envy within their circles of influence. They think of themselves as helping mothers and babies through acts of humble service. The suggestion that they are instead leading women down a path of deception, danger, and risk of grave injury and death is completely unbearable. It threatens everything they know and believe about themselves.

It is no surprise that few midwives allow themselves this rude awakening. For me to come to terms with my role in this culture of deception, I had to be willing to walk away from a million-dollar business, a career, my credentials, and my position of respect in the world of midwifery. I had to put most of my social connections and friendships, both close and casual, on the line, not knowing how well they would fare, or if they would survive at all. I had to question my own sense of self, my concept of who I was and my place in the world, and be willing to start over again.

Yet, we have to be willing to do that difficult work. Human nature may lead us to make great errors, but it is our responsibility to do what we can to overcome them and to set things right. I know that decisions I have made have hurt people, a fact that causes me great dissonance because they are people I genuinely care about. Some of them are reading this right now. *I'm sorry for what I did, which was wrong, and which caused you pain.*

It took me longer than I'd like to admit. I took my time buying gasoline and matches. I lingered while saying goodbye to some bridges, running my fingers lovingly over the handrails, admiring the beauty I still saw in them. I took a deep breath, lit a match, and watched as the flame burned closer and closer to my fingers, and blew it out. I took out another match, and watched as that hot flash of truth slowly got closer to my fingers, and blew it out again. I lit one last match, held it tight, and witnessed its slow progress down toward my hand. Just before that moment when it surely would have burned me, I dropped it. And here I am. And that blaze, that fiery blaze roaring before me, it is more beautiful than the bridges that it burns.

References

Ackermann-Liebrich, U., Voegeli, T., Gunter-Witt, K., Kunz, I., Zullig, M., Schindler, C., Maurer, M., & Zurich Study Team. (1996). Home versus hospital deliveries: follow up study of matched pairs for procedures and outcome. *BMJ*, 313(7068), 1313-1318.

Amelink-Verburg, M. P., Verloove-Vanhorick, S. P., Hakkenberg, R. M., Veldhuijzen, I. M., Bennebroek Gravenhorst, J., & Buitendijk, S. E. (2008). Evaluation of 280,000 cases in Dutch midwifery practices: A descriptive study. *British Journal of Obstetrics and Gynecology*, 115(5), 570-578.

Anderson, R. E. & Murphy, P. A. (1995). Outcomes of 11,788 planned home births attended by certified nurse-midwives: A retrospective descriptive study. *Journal of Nurse Midwifery*, 40(6), 483-492.

Birthplace in England Collaborative Group. (2011). Perinatal and maternal outcomes by planned place of birth for healthy women with low risk pregnancies: the Birthplace in England national prospective cohort study. *BMJ*, 343:d7400.

Chamberlain, G., Wraight, A., & Crowley, P. (Eds.). (1997). *Home births: The report of the 1994 confidential*

enquiry by the National Birthday Trust Fund.
Lancaster, UK: Parthenon Publishing Group Ltd.

Cheng, Y.W., Snowden, J.M., King, T.L., & Caughey, A.B. (2013). Selected perinatal outcomes associated with planned home births in the United States. *American Journal of Obstetrics and Gynecology, 209*(4), 325.e1-8.

Cheyney, M., Bovbjerg, M., Everson, C., Gordon, W., Hannibal, D., & Vedam, S. (2014). Outcomes of care for 16,924 planned home births in the United States: the Midwives Alliance of North America statistics project, 2004 to 2009. *Journal of Midwifery & Women's Health, 59*, 17-27.

Cawthon, L. (1996). *Planned home births: Outcomes among Medicaid women in Washington State.* Olympia, WA: Washington Department of Social and Health Services.

de Jonge, A., van der Goes, B. Y., Ravelli, A. C., Amelink-Verburg, M. P., Mol, B. W., Nijhuis, J. G., Bennebroek Gravenhorst, J., & Buitendijk, S. E. (2009). Perinatal mortality and morbidity in a nationwide cohort of 529,688 low-risk planned home and hospital births. *British Journal of Obstetrics and Gynecology, 116*(9), 1177-1184.

Declercq, E., MacDorman, M. F., Menacker, F., & Stotland, N. (2010). Characteristics of planned and unplanned home births in 19 states. *Obstetrics & Gynecology*, 116(1), 93-99.

Dowswell, T., Thornton, J. G., Hewison, J., Lilford, R. J., Raisler, J., Macfarlane, A., Young, G., Newburn, M., Dodds, R. & Settatree, R. S. (1996). Should there be a trial of home versus hospital delivery in the United Kingdom? Measuring outcomes other than safety is feasible. *BMJ*, 312(7033), 753-757.

Evers, A.C.C., Brouwers, H.A.A., Hukkelhoven, C.W.P.M., Nikkels, P.G.J., Boon, J., van Egmond-Linden, A., Hillegersberg, J., Snuif, Y.S., Sterken-Hooisma, S., Bruinse, H.W., & Kwee, A. (2010). Perinatal mortality and severe morbidity in low and high risk term pregnancies in the Netherlands: prospective cohort study. *BMJ*, 341, c5639.

Grunebaum, A., McCullough, L.B., Sapra, K.J., Brent, R.L., Levene, M.I., Arabin, B., & Chervenak, F.A. (2013). Apgar score of 0 at 5 minutes and neonatal seizures or serious neurologic dysfunction in relation to birth setting. *American Journal of Obstetrics and Gynecology*, 209(323), e1-6.

Gulbransen, G., Hilton, J., McKay, L., & Cox, A. (1997). Home birth in New Zealand 1973-93: Incidence and mortality. *New Zealand Medical Journal*, 110(1040), 87-89.

Hendrix, M., Van Horck, M., Moreta, D., Nieman, F., Nieuwenhuijze, M., Severens, J., & Nijhuis, J. (2009). Why women do not accept randomisation for place of birth: feasibility of a RCT in The Netherlands. *British Journal of Obstetrics and Gynecology*, 116(4), 537-544.

Hutton, E. K., Reitsma, A. H., & Kaufman, K. (2009). Outcomes associated with planned home and planned hospital births in low-risk women attended by midwives in Ontario, Canada, 2003-2006: A retrospective cohort study. *Birth: Issues in Perinatal Care*, 36(3), 180-189.

Janssen, P. A., Saxell, L., Page, L. A., Klein, M. C., Liston, R. M., & Lee, S. K. (2009). Outcomes of planned home births with registered midwife versus planned hospital birth with midwife or physician. *Canadian Medical Association Journal*, 181(6-7), 377-383.

Janssen, P. A., Lee, S. K., Ryan, E. M., Etches, D. J., Farquharson, D. F., Peacock, D., & Klein, M. C. (2002). Outcomes of planned home births versus planned hospital births after regulation of midwifery in British Columbia. *Canadian Medical Association Journal*, 166(3), 315-323.

Janssen, P. (2002, June 11). The pleasures of home birth? [Letters]. *Canadian Medical Association Journal*, 166(12), 1511.

Johnson, K. C., & Daviss, B. A. (2005). Outcomes of planned home birth with certified professional midwives: large prospective study in North America. *BMJ*, 330, 1416.

Kennare, R. M., Keirse, M. J., Tucker, G. R., & Chan, A. C. (2009). Planned home and hospital births in South Australia 1991-2006: differences in outcomes. *Medical Journal of Australia*, 192(2), 76-80.

Lake, R. (2011, June 26). Mothers deserve options. *Huffington Post*. Retrieved from http://www.huffingtonpost.com/ricki-lake/mothers-deserve-options_b_884900.html

Leslie, M.S., & Romano, A. (2007). Appendix: Birth can safely take place at home and in birthing centers. *Journal of Perinatal Education*, 16(Supplement 1):81S-88S. doi:10.1624/105812407X173236

MacDorman, M. F., Declercq, E., & Menacker, F. (2011). Trends and characteristics of home births in the

United States by race and ethnicity, 1990-2006. *Birth: Issues in Perinatal Care,* 38(1):17-23.

Murphy, P. A. & Fullerton, J. (1998). Outcomes of intended home births in nurse-midwifery practice: A prospective descriptive study. *Obstetrics & Gynecology*, 92(3), 461-470.

Northern Region Perinatal Mortality Survey Coordinating Group. (1996). Collaborative survey of perinatal loss in planned and unplanned home births. *BMJ,* 313(7068), 1306-1309.

Olsen, O., & Clausen, J. A. (2012). Planned hospital birth versus planned home birth. *Cochrane Database of Systematic Reviews*, doi: 10.1002/14651858.CD000352.pub2.

Olsen, O. (1997). Meta-analysis of the safety of home birth. *Birth: Issues in Perinatal Care,* 24(1), 4-13.

Rooks, J. (2013). Untitled letter to the Oregon State Legislature. Retrieved from https://olis.leg.state.or.us/liz/2013R1/Downloads/Com mittee MeetingDocument/8585

Schlenzka, P.F. (1999). Safety of alternative approaches to childbirth [Unpublished Dissertation]. Palo Alto, CA: Department of Sociology, Stanford University.

Tavris, C., & Aronson, E. (2007). *Mistakes were made (But not by me)*. New York, NY: Houghton Mifflin Harcourt Publishing Company.

United States Department of Health and Human Services (US DHHS), Centers for Disease Control and Prevention (CDC), National Center for Health Statistics (NCHS), Division of Vital Statistics, Natality public-use data 2007-2013, on CDC WONDER Online Database. (2015 January). Accessed at http://wonder.cdc.gov/natality-current.html on Feb 8, 2015 9:32:09 PM

van der Kooy, J., Poeran, J., de Graff, J. P., Birnie, E., Denktass, S., Steegers, E. A. P., & Bonsel, G. J. (2011). Planned home compared with planned hospital births in the Netherlands: intrapartum and early neonatal death in low-risk pregnancies. *Obstetrics & Gynecology,* 118(5), 1037-1046.

Vedam, S., Schummers, L., Stoll, K., & Fulton, C. (2012). Home birth: an annotated guide to the literature. *MANA.org.* Retrieved from http://mana.org/research/section-a-best-available-studies-grouped-by-design-level-of-evidence

Wasden, S., Perlman, J., Chasen, S., & Lipkind, H. (2014). 506: Home birth and risk of neonatal hypoxic ischemic encephalopathy. *American Journal of Obstetrics & Gynecology*, 210(1), S251.

Wiegers, T. A., Keirse, M. J., van der Zee, J., & Berghs, G. A. (1996). Outcome of planned home and planned hospital births in low risk pregnancies: prospective study in midwifery practices in the Netherlands. *BMJ*, 313, 1309-1313.

For more information, charts, and updates, visit
www.honestmidwife.com

Follow at www.facebook.com/honestmidwife